HERBAL REMEDIES FOR PSORIATIC ARTHRITIS

Empower Your Journey To Wellness With Herbs For Alleviating Pain, Restoring Joint Health And Nurturing Overall Well-Being

DR. CARDEN KYRIE

DISCLAIMER

The only goal of this book is informational. Every effort has been taken by the author and publisher to ensure that the information provided is accurate. But the material in this book is given "as is," without any express or implied representation, warranty, or condition as to its accuracy, completeness, or suitability for any particular purpose.

Any loss, damage, or injury resulting from using the information in this book, or from any action or decision made as a result of such use, will not be covered by the author's or publisher's liability. It is recommended that readers seek the assistance of a certified specialist for guidance specific to their situation.

The opinions and viewpoints conveyed in this book belong to the author and may not necessarily represent the official stance or policies of any specified organizations or people. Any likeness to real-life occurrences, places, or people—living or deceased—is wholly coincidental.

No specific product, service, or therapy discussed in this book is endorsed by the author or publisher. Any reference to goods or services is made only for informative reasons and is not intended as a recommendation or endorsement.

Before making any judgments or acting on any information, readers are urged to independently confirm it all. Any unfavorable effects or repercussions arising from the usage of the material included in this book are disclaimed by the author and publisher.

By using this book, you consent to absolving the publisher and author of any and all claims, obligations, or losses resulting from your use of the material in it.

I appreciate your cooperation and understanding.

TABLE OF CONTENTS

CHAPTER ONE

INTRODUCTION TO PSORIATIC ARTHRITIS

PSORIATIC ARTHRITIS OVERVIEW

People who have already been diagnosed with psoriasis, a skin illness marked by red, scaly patches, may also develop Psoriatic Arthritis (PsA), a chronic inflammatory condition. Psoriatic arthritis affects the joints as well as the skin, resulting in pain, stiffness, and swelling. It falls under the category of autoimmune disease, in which inflammation results from the immune system of the body unintentionally attacking healthy cells and tissues. Psoriatic arthritis affects a considerable proportion of people with psoriasis, while its prevalence varies. The ailment may present in diverse ways, impacting joints on either side or both, and its intensity may vary from moderate to severe. People with psoriatic arthritis encounter difficulties navigating the complexity of a chronic, multifaceted ailment that not only affects their physical health but also their emotional and psychological well-being.

THE VALUE OF HERBAL TREATMENTS

Herbal treatments have gained popularity as an alternate method of treating several illnesses, including psoriatic arthritis. Herbal medicines are significant because they can reduce inflammation, alleviate symptoms, and enhance general health. Herbal therapies, in contrast to conventional drugs, frequently incorporate traditional knowledge and employ plants and natural substances as means of addressing health issues. This method, which emphasizes the connection between the physical, mental, and emotional elements of health, is in line with the growing interest in complementary and holistic medicine. Examining the historical background of herbal medicine, the wide variety of plants with alleged medicinal benefits, and the empirical data substantiating their effectiveness are necessary to comprehend the significance of herbal remedies in the treatment of psoriatic arthritis.

Numerous plants and botanical extracts with anti-inflammatory and immunomodulatory qualities are used in herbal treatments for psoriatic arthritis. These organic ingredients might aid in the general management of the ailment in addition to reducing joint pain and inflammation. Because herbal therapies are holistic, they take into account not only the symptoms of psoriatic arthritis but also the underlying reasons that contribute to its development and progression. It is important to investigate these cures from a nuanced standpoint, keeping in mind that individual differences in their effectiveness may occur and that they may be used in addition to traditional treatments.

We examine the complex interplay among the immune system, inflammation, and joint health in this discussion on psoriatic arthritis and the value of herbal treatments. Understanding how Psoriatic Arthritis affects a person's quality of life highlights the necessity of a thorough and individualized management strategy. We seek to understand the possible advantages of using herbal remedies, as well as the cultural and historical relevance of traditional medicine and the changing face of integrative healthcare. This introduction lays the groundwork for a more thorough examination of the complexities of psoriatic arthritis and the potential benefits of herbal medicines for improving the health of those who are afflicted.

CHAPTER TWO

KNOWLEDGE OF PSORIATIC ARTHRITIS

PSORIATIC ARTHRITIS: WHAT IS IT?

Skin and joints are both impacted by the long-term inflammatory disease known as psoriatic arthritis (PsA). It is categorized as an autoimmune illness, meaning inflammation results from the immune system of the body accidentally attacking its tissues. Psoriasis, a skin disorder marked by red, scaly areas, is intimately linked to psoriatic arthritis. The relationship between Psoriasis and arthritis in PsA suggests that the immune system plays a role in both diseases. Psoriatic arthritis usually develops in people who have psoriasis already, though joint symptoms can appear before or at the same time as the skin symptoms.

REASONS AND DANGER ELEMENTS

Although the precise origins of psoriatic arthritis remain unclear, a confluence of immunological, environmental, and genetic variables is thought to have a role in the disease's development. A person's genetic susceptibility is important since those who have a family history of PsA or psoriasis are more susceptible. HLA-B27 is one gene that has been linked to a higher risk of developing psoriatic arthritis. In people with a genetic predisposition, environmental events including infections or accidents might cause PsA to develop. Psoriatic arthritis is primarily caused by an aberrant immune response, more precisely an excessive inflammatory response.

SIGNS AND PROGNOSIS

There is a wide range of symptoms associated with psoriatic arthritis that can impact various body areas. Common symptoms include stiffness, edema, and discomfort in the joints; psoriasis skin signs are frequently present as well. The fingers, toes, knees, and spine joints are the most frequently impacted. Entheses are the regions where tendons or ligaments join to bones; psoriatic arthritis can also affect these sites, resulting in enthesitis. Diagnosis might be difficult because symptoms can vary greatly in intensity and course from person to person.

A thorough assessment of the patient's symptoms, medical history, and physical examination are necessary for the diagnosis of psoriatic arthritis. One important sign is the existence of skin lesions associated with psoriasis, as well as joint pain and inflammation. Joint inflammation and injury can be evaluated with imaging tests including magnetic resonance imaging (MRI) and X-rays. Blood tests can also be used to measure inflammation markers including erythrocyte sedimentation rate (ESR) and C-reactive protein (CRP) and to rule out other forms of arthritis. Working together to treat both the joint and skin components, rheumatologists and dermatologists are frequently needed to reach a definitive diagnosis.

TRADITIONAL THERAPY CHOICES

The goals of traditional Psoriatic Arthritis treatment are to reduce inflammation, manage symptoms, and shield the joints from harm. NSAIDs, or nonsteroidal anti-inflammatory medicines, are frequently recommended to treat inflammation and relieve pain. Methotrexate is one of the disease-modifying antirheumatic medications (DMARDs) used to decrease the course of joint deterioration. A more recent class of drugs called biologics targets particular immune system components that contribute to inflammation. TNF-alpha inhibitors and IL-17 inhibitors are two medications that have demonstrated effectiveness in treating the symptoms of psoriatic arthritis. Corticosteroids can also be used to temporarily relieve severe symptoms.

Psoriatic arthritis is a complicated inflammatory disease that closely resembles psoriasis and presents as joint inflammation. Its development is influenced by several factors, including genetic, environmental, and immunological ones, however, its precise causes are yet unknown.

CHAPTER THREE

THE FUNCTION OF HERBAL TREATMENTS HISTORICAL ANGLE

The traditional uses of herbal treatments date back many centuries and are ingrained in the traditions of many different countries. Herbs and plants have long been valued for their therapeutic qualities, serving as the cornerstone of traditional medical practices throughout human history. Herbs have been used for thousands of years in traditional Chinese medicine and Ayurveda in India. The historical viewpoint emphasizes how closely humans are related to the plant kingdom and how dependent we are on nature's abundance to keep us well and heal our illnesses.

BASIS OF HERBAL MEDICINE SCIENCE

The complex biochemistry of plants and their possible therapeutic benefits are explored in the scientific study of herbal remedies. Numerous herbs have active ingredients that interact with the body to affect physiological functions. Sophisticated methodologies are used in modern research to discover and comprehend these bioactive components. Herbs' synergistic combination of chemicals typically contributes to their therapeutic effectiveness. Furthermore, pharmacology and molecular biology developments have made it possible for researchers to decipher the workings of herbal treatments, giving them a scientific foundation for their traditional efficacy.

ADVANTAGES AND DRAWBACKS OF HERBAL TREATMENTS

Herbal treatments have a wide range of advantages, from little symptomatic relief to significant therapeutic outcomes. Herbal medicine's holistic approach, which frequently treats the underlying cause of an illness rather than just its symptoms, is one of its main benefits. Furthermore, compared to many synthetic medications, herbs are typically seen to be safer and have fewer adverse effects. But it's important to recognize the limitations. Herbal product standardization can be difficult, resulting in differences in efficacy and potency. Furthermore, in acute cases where prompt intervention is crucial, the gradual onset of action and the requirement for persistent administration may provide difficulties.

COMBINING TRADITIONAL MEDICAL PROCEDURES WITH HERBAL THERAPIES

A developing trend in healthcare is the combination of herbal remedies with traditional medicine, which emphasizes a complementary approach. By recognizing the advantages of both modalities, this integration seeks to maximize therapeutic outcomes through a synergistic impact. Herbal therapies can help improve general well-being, control chronic diseases, and reduce the negative effects of conventional medications. Healthcare practitioners must, however, proceed cautiously with this integration, taking patient preferences, possible herb-drug interactions, and the requirement for evidence-based treatments into account. To promote a complete and patient-centered approach to healing that incorporates the best aspects of both ancient wisdom and contemporary medical science, cooperation between herbalists and conventional healthcare specialists is imperative.

The role of herbal remedies is complex, has a long history, is backed by an increasing amount of scientific research, and is becoming more and more accepted in contemporary healthcare paradigms alongside conventional treatments. A more knowledgeable and comprehensive approach to incorporating herbal remedies into modern healthcare practices is made possible by having a thorough understanding of the scientific foundations, the historical background, and the subtle advantages and limitations.

CHAPTER FOUR

FREQUENTLY USED HERBS FOR PSORIATIC ARTHRITIS

TURMERIC & CURCUMIN

Curcumin, a spice derived from the Curcuma longa plant, is one of the most extensively researched and well-known herbs for treating psoriatic arthritis. Curcumin, the primary ingredient in turmeric, has anti-inflammatory qualities. Curcumin may lessen psoriatic arthritis symptoms by lowering inflammation and adjusting the immune system, according to research. According to certain studies, curcumin can block specific inflammatory pathways, which can help people with psoriatic arthritis-related joint stiffness and pain.

GINGER

Another popular spice that has shown anti-inflammatory and antioxidant properties, ginger may help those with psoriatic arthritis. Bioactive substances found in ginger, such as gingerol, have been demonstrated to have anti-inflammatory qualities. Psoriatic arthritis-related joint pain and inflammation may be lessened by including ginger in the diet or taking it as a supplement. But before incorporating large amounts of ginger into the diet, especially for people with pre-existing medical disorders or on medication, it is imperative to speak with a healthcare provider.

BOSWELLIA SERRATA

Known by most as Indian frankincense, Boswellia serrata is a herb with anti-inflammatory qualities that has long been utilized in Ayurvedic medicine. Boswellic acids, the active ingredients in boswellia, have the potential to lessen inflammation by blocking specific enzymes that contribute to the inflammatory process. According to certain research, Boswellia serrata extract may be useful in treating joint stiffness and pain associated with arthritis. As with any herbal supplement, it's important to speak with a healthcare professional to figure out the right dosage and make sure it won't conflict with other prescriptions.

WILLOW BARK

For millennia, people have utilized willow bark as a home treatment to relieve pain and inflammation. Salicin, a substance comparable to aspirin's active component, is present in it. Willow bark may help people with psoriatic arthritis because it is thought to have analgesic and anti-inflammatory properties. Although there is little few research on willow bark specifically for psoriatic arthritis, historical usage and anecdotal evidence point to the possibility that it could provide pain relief for joints. Willow bark should always be used under a doctor's supervision, just like any other herbal therapy, especially for people who have allergies or sensitivity issues.

ALOE VERA

Known for its anti-inflammatory and wound-healing qualities, aloe vera is a succulent plant that is occasionally used to treat psoriatic arthritis-related skin complaints.

Aloe vera can be administered topically to relieve skin irritation and encourage healing, while its effectiveness in treating joint complaints is not as well-established. Aloe vera gel or lotion can help some people with psoriatic arthritis with skin-related problems. It is imperative, therefore, to select pure, high-quality aloe vera products and seek medical advice before applying them to afflicted regions.

OTHER HERBAL OPTIONS

Several other herbs are being investigated for their possible advantages in treating psoriatic arthritis in addition to the ones already listed. These could include, among other things, stinging nettle, green tea, and cat's claw. The woody vine from which a cat's claw is grown is prized for its anti-inflammatory qualities. Stinging nettle has long been utilized for its anti-inflammatory qualities, and green tea possesses antioxidant-rich polyphenols. Even though these herbs may help some people, it's crucial to use caution while using them and speak with a healthcare provider to be sure they're safe and effective. This is especially important when using them in addition to traditional therapies for psoriatic arthritis. Integrative methods, which incorporate herbal therapies with medical advice, may provide a more comprehensive approach to treating psoriatic arthritis symptoms.

CHAPTER FIVE

RECIPES AND FORMULATIONS USING HERBS

HERBAL INFUSIONS AND TEAS

For millennia, people from many different cultures have valued herbal teas and infusions for their calming and healing qualities. These drinks are made by steeping fresh or dried herbs in hot water to release their active ingredients into the drink. Herbs come in a broad variety, each with their own distinct tastes and health advantages.

Herbal teas, which come in soothing flavors like chamomile and energizing peppermint, are not only a fun way to stay hydrated but may also be used as a natural cure for a variety of illnesses. Herbal teas are made by carefully selecting plant components, such as leaves, flowers, or roots, and steeping them for the ideal amount of time to maximize the extraction of medicinal chemicals.

EXTRACTS AND TINCTURES

Herbal treatments in concentrated forms such as tinctures and extracts are made from plants and use alcohol, glycerin, or vinegar to extract the therapeutic qualities of the plants. Tinctures are a quick and effective approach to using herbal medicine since this process allows for a high concentration of the herb's active ingredients.

The plant material is macerated and steeped in the selected solvent as part of the extraction process. Tinctures are a convenient choice for people who want to benefit from herbal medicines without having to consume significant amounts of plant material because of their lengthy shelf life and ease of dosage control. Tinctures are a powerful and practical substitute for conventional herbal treatments, whether utilized for immune support, stress alleviation, or other health issues.

TOPICAL APPLICATIONS AND POULTICES

Herbs can be externally applied as poultices or topical applications to treat a variety of skin ailments, wounds, or localized discomfort. Generally, a poultice is made by combining ground or crushed herbs with a liquid to create a paste, which is then applied directly to the area that is afflicted. By directly absorbing the herb's active ingredients through the skin, this technique facilitates healing and reduces discomfort. Because of their calming and anti-inflammatory qualities, herbs including comfrey, calendula, and aloe vera are frequently used in poultices. Herbal creams, salves, and oils are other well-liked topical treatments that offer a quick and focused way to treat joint discomfort, muscle aches, and skin problems.

SUPPLEMENTS WITH HERBS

A wide range of goods are referred to as herbal supplements, and their purpose is to enhance general health and well-being by introducing the health benefits of medicinal plants into one's diet. These supplements could be in the shape of pills, liquid extracts, powders, or capsules. The choice of herbs in these mixtures is frequently dictated by the scientific evidence substantiating their effectiveness as well as their traditional use. Herbal remedies for digestive health, stress reduction, and immunological support are common. Herbal supplements have the advantage of being convenient, having consistent dosages, and having the capacity to blend different herbs to address different health issues. But to guarantee safety and effectiveness, pick premium supplements and speak with a medical professional.

DIETARY AND LIFESTYLE FACTORS ANTI-INFLAMMATORY DIET

An anti-inflammatory diet is a comprehensive nutritional strategy that aims to lessen the body's inflammatory response. Numerous medical diseases, including diabetes, autoimmune illnesses, and heart disease, have been connected to chronic inflammation.

Eating foods that reduce inflammation and avoiding those that exacerbate it is the fundamental tenet of an anti-inflammatory diet.

Omega-3 fatty acid-rich foods include walnuts, flaxseeds, and fatty fish, which are well-known for their anti-inflammatory qualities. Rich in phytochemicals and antioxidants, colorful fruits and vegetables are also essential in the fight against inflammation. Leafy greens, cruciferous veggies, and berries are great options. An anti-inflammatory diet can also benefit from including healthy fats like olive oil and favoring whole grains over refined grains.

Conversely, red meat overindulgence, processed foods, and sugary drinks have all been linked to elevated levels of inflammation. People can proactively reduce inflammation with their diet by prioritizing nutrient-dense, whole foods and reducing processed and refined options.

PHYSICAL ACTIVITY AND EXERCISE

Physical activity and regular exercise are essential parts of a healthy lifestyle. Apart from the widely acknowledged advantages of maintaining a healthy weight and cardiovascular system, physical activity has a significant effect on psychological health. Endorphins are naturally occurring mood enhancers that are released when you exercise, lowering stress and anxiety. In addition, it helps with sleep, enhances cognitive performance, and improves general quality of life.

Exercise regimens and intensities might change depending on personal preferences and fitness levels. Strength training improves bone density and muscle tone, while aerobic activities like cycling, jogging, and walking strengthen the heart. Pilates and yoga are examples of flexibility activities that increase joint mobility and lower the chance of injury.

Even more advantageous than scheduled exercise sessions might be making physical activity a part of everyday activities. Examples include walking briskly during breaks or using the stairs rather than the elevator. The secret is to choose sustainable and pleasurable activities that will encourage a long-term dedication to an active lifestyle.

TECHNIQUES FOR STRESS MANAGEMENT

In the fast-paced world of today, preserving mental and physical well-being requires effective stress management. To lessen the negative effects of stress on the body and mind, a variety of stress management strategies can be used. Deep breathing exercises and guided meditation sessions are two examples of mindfulness and meditation techniques that are well known for their capacity to induce calm and lower stress levels.

Taking part in joyful and fulfilling hobbies and activities can serve as a potent diversion from the stresses of everyday life. Engaging in pleasurable activities, such as reading, gardening, or practicing a musical instrument, offers a psychological reprieve and a feeling of achievement.

A key element of stress management is understanding when to say "no" and setting up healthy limits. Overwhelming feelings can be avoided by prioritizing things, dividing them into manageable chunks, and refraining from overcommitting.

Another essential component of stress management is social support. Having and preserving close relationships with friends and family offers a priceless emotional safety net in trying times. Furthermore, as was already said, engaging in regular physical activity is a powerful way to decrease stress.

A comprehensive approach to lifestyle and nutritional choices entails the adoption of an anti-inflammatory diet, consistent exercise and physical activity, and the application of efficient stress management strategies. Together, these components support general health—both mental and physical—and help people lead balanced, satisfying lives.

CHAPTER SIX

SAFETY MEASURES AND POTENTIAL REPERCUSSIONS

CONSULTING WITH MEDICAL EXPERTS

Speaking with medical experts is one of the most important safety measures to take while making any decisions about one's health. Consult with licensed healthcare providers before beginning any new therapy, medication, or supplement program. This is especially crucial because the safety and effectiveness of therapies can be significantly impacted by a person's medical history, current drugs, and specific health problems. Healthcare providers are qualified to evaluate these variables and offer tailored advice so that the treatment plan selected is in line with the patient's overall health profile.

POSSIBLE DRUG INTERACTIONS

To avoid side effects and guarantee the best possible treatment results, it is essential to comprehend possible drug interactions. Whether they are over-the-counter pharmaceuticals, herbal supplements, or prescription drugs, some chemicals can interact with one another in ways that reduce their efficacy or cause unwanted side effects. Combining drugs, for example, may increase or decrease the intended effects of each drug, endangering the patient's health. To prevent and manage potential drug interactions, people should fully disclose to their healthcare professionals all of their medication history, including any supplements or alternative therapies.

SAFETY PRECAUTIONS AND MONITORING

These two elements are essential to reducing the dangers connected to any medical intervention. Healthcare providers can monitor a patient's progress with a medicine or treatment and make necessary adjustments regularly. It also makes it easier to identify negative interactions or reactions early on, allowing for timely intervention. Respecting the recommended dosages, frequency, and length of therapy, together with any particular instructions given by medical specialists, are all part of the safety precautions. This entails being aware of any adverse effects and reporting any unusual symptoms or concerns right away. It could also be advised to undergo regular check-ups and laboratory testing to make sure the medication is safe and effective over time.

In the field of healthcare, the significance of speaking with medical specialists, identifying possible drug interactions, and putting monitoring and safety measures in place cannot be emphasized. Together, these safety measures make up an all-encompassing strategy for patient care, guaranteeing that therapies are customized to meet specific needs, reduce risks, and maximize therapeutic advantages. People can confidently and under the supervision of trained healthcare professionals navigate their health journeys by following these well-informed and cautious procedures.

FIRST-HAND ACCOUNTS OF HERBAL MEDICINE USE

Individuals' personal experiences with herbal medicines differ greatly from one another since reactions to these natural compounds can be impacted by a variety of circumstances, including individual sensitivities, pre-existing medical issues, and general health. Herbal medicines are often used to treat a variety of health issues, but it's important to use caution and be aware of any potential conflicts with other medications or medical problems.

The fact that herbal treatments are not subject to the same regulations as pharmaceutical drugs is an important factor to take into account. Variations in the efficacy and safety of herbal medications may result from this lack of consistency in composition and dosage. Experiences with herbal medicines firsthand frequently emphasize how crucial it is to speak with medical specialists before implementing any new remedies into one's routine, particularly if one is on prescription medications or managing a chronic disease.

There may be hazards associated with natural treatments and prescription drugs. For example, some herbs can affect how well medications are absorbed, metabolized, or eliminated, which might change how effective they are or result in unanticipated adverse effects. Anecdotes from personal experience frequently highlight the necessity for people to be transparent with their healthcare professionals regarding the use of herbal treatments to guarantee a thorough awareness of any potential interactions.

Furthermore, firsthand accounts emphasize how important it is to understand that various people will respond differently to herbal medicines. A person may not have the same results from something that works well for them. The various outcomes seen are a result of differences in genetic makeup, lifestyle choices, and individual health status. People who relate their experiences frequently emphasize how crucial it is, to begin with moderate doses and keep an eye on how their bodies respond to herbal medicines, particularly when attempting them for the first time.

The cumulative effects of herbal therapies must also be taken into account, particularly when utilizing many products at once. Personal accounts frequently highlight the necessity of exercising caution and introducing new treatments gradually to reduce the possibility of negative reactions. In these cases, regular discussion with healthcare practitioners becomes essential to ensure a thorough awareness of potential interactions between various herbal therapies and conventional treatments.

Notwithstanding the potential advantages of herbal medicines, firsthand accounts highlight the significance of being aware of any adverse responses or side effects. People who share their experiences generally emphasize how different allergic reactions might be from one another and how important it is to seek medical assistance as soon as possible if any negative reactions arise. This highlights how important it is for each person to keep an eye on their health and recognize any warning signals that can point to the need for professional medical assistance.

Finally, personal experiences with herbal remedies highlight the significance of using caution and awareness when utilizing these natural treatments. Including herbal medicines in one's routine for health and wellness requires careful consideration of individual responses, education about possible drug interactions, and consultation with healthcare specialists.